Poison Ivy,
Pets, & People

*Scratching the Poison Ivy,
Oak, and Sumac Itch*

Another book from the
10 things to know™
series, companion to

Poison Ivy, Pets & People
*Scratching the Poison Ivy, Oak,
and Sumac Itch*

_____

Bees & Other Stinging Insects
BEE Aware and *BEE* Safe!

_____

Poison Ivy, Pets, & People

Scratching the Poison Ivy, Oak, and Sumac Itch

Heidi Ratner-Connolly
and
Randy Connolly

P Prevent with Knowledge

L Learn to Identify

A Avoid Conscienciously

N Naturally Eliminate When Possible

T Treat Symptomatically and Safely

Athens County
Library Services
Nelsonville, Ohio

Book Design by Heidi Ratner-Connolly
ISBN 0-9722400-1-2
Published by 2LAKES PUBLISHING
Distributed by IPG/Chicago Review Press

Randy and I would love to hear about any of your per-
sonalized best remedies and treatments for poison ivy.
When we update our book, we will try to add in your
suggestions.

Please email us at:
heidi@2lakespublishing.com
randy@2lakespublishing.com

Please note: This book is written for informational purposes only. The treatments mentioned herein are examples of treatments we have found useful or have been suggested by others. If you have come in contact with poison ivy, oak, or sumac, or with someone/something that has, please use common sense when treating and consult with a health care provider. The treatment options herein should not be considered viable options for everyone and should always be discussed with your health care provider before use.

Acknowledgments:

We would like to say a special thank you to Martha Tenney, our friend and editor extraordinaire, who helped us put this book in order and bring it to its current state of fruition.

When Heidi Ratner-Connolly and Randy Connolly found themselves frustrated by the lack of down-to-earth, accessible information on topics that were of particular personal concern, they decided to write their own books to answer that need. It was then that

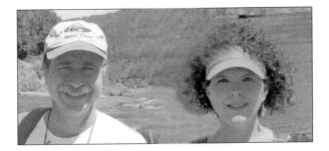

2LAKES PUBLISHING and the 10 things to know™ series of books were born, generating books that are always *long on information when you're short on time.* The Connollys are dedicated to publishing books that help people live healthier, happier lives, and to living their own lives in the pursuit of a similar goal. They are currently living on the magnificant coast of Oregon.

CONTENTS

The 5th Thing You Need to Know

The 6th Thing You Need to Know

The 7th Thing You Need to Know

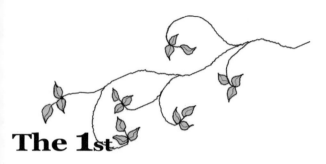

The 1st

Thing to Know

Scratching the Poison Ivy, Oak, and Sumac Itch

It's a Jungle Out There

It's time to face the facts: **It's a jungle out there.** Especially when it comes to dealing with poison ivy,* oak, or sumac.

If you're anything like my husband or me, you know what we're talking about: the dreaded and feared ivy vine that goes anywhere, climbs anything and stays for what seems like forever just to make your every waking moment sheer misery! We've heard many horrific stories; here is our own.

*Unless we indicate otherwise, wherever we have written *poison ivy*, *oak* or *sumac*, can be inserted, or we refer to all three as *"the trio."*

When Randy was just a kid, not more than seven years old, he was playing baseball in a park. Nearby, a neighbor decided to burn brush and leaves on a typical, sunny, May, New England day. Randy inhaled poison ivy oil from the smoke and ended up staying over two weeks in the hospital. He almost died there, and ever since then his allergy to poison ivy has been instant and violent.

So, you can imagine the fear it holds for us, and how far we might go to avoid it. We have a beautiful golden retriever who is probably the friendliest dog in the universe. (I won't regale you with stories here, that he retrieves nothing he can't eat, and will make friends with any human who offers him something to eat.) Naturally, we love walking with our dog, especially by the ocean where we live, and we were surprised—and not too happy—to learn that poison ivy also loves the seashore more often than not.

That means our dog, Dakota, spends more time on his leash than we'd like so he's less likely to mix it up with other "free-roaming" dogs who may have roamed through poison ivy, and also so he is less likely to roam through it himself. We end up trying to avoid his mingling with other dogs most of the year. Not only is this difficult, we feel bad about doing it. And, of course, it's not entirely possible either, so we have become well versed in cleansing methods for humans and animals alike. When other animals come a callin', we go a washin'.

We are careful in other people's homes and have a high level of suspicion around animals we don't know and/or homes we don't know. Sometimes we don't even sit down. And we're always washing our hands. About this time, I can hear you say, *"These people are truly paranoid…we could never be that obsessive."* But here's the payoff. Though our whole family is excruciatingly allergic to poison ivy, none of us has gotten it in years!

What else do we do? We worry about handling our son's baseball—after all, who knows where it's been? Experiencing nature is a favorite activity of ours, so hiking means staying on a **wide** path, and definitely not through dense foliage. Gardening is done very carefully, if at all. Sure puts a crimp in our style, I can tell you. But the good news is that with enough of the right kind of knowledge you can live a perfectly "normal" life. Go ahead: hike, camp, garden and romp—as long as you really know how to identify, and avoid poison ivy, oak or sumac, you should be able to partake in any activities you enjoy without fear of imminent danger.

You might assume, at this point, that we are pretty well read on this subject; we have, in fact, collected files of information for many years. But we decided that updating our knowledge could help all of us stay a little more current on the facts, so that together we might be able to stay on top of one of Mother Nature's greatest plant world challenges.

So, here are the facts, from the best of our research. May this book be of service to you, and may you never come in contact with this ghoulish greenery again!

And always remember:

**Identification
and Avoidance
are the
ONLY Real Means
of Prevention!**

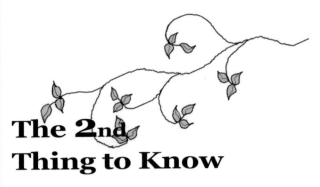

The 2nd Thing to Know

The Real Scoop on Poison Ivy, Oak, and Sumac

Myth or Reality?

One of the big problems with poison ivy is that we've all heard so many stories about how people have gotten it, how long it's lasted, how contagious it is, etc., that we don't really know what's myth and what's reality. After you've read this book, you should feel confident that you know, once and for all *all* the in's and out's, and that you will have gotten *everything you need to know* to scratch the poison ivy, oak, and sumac itch.

Another one of the problems with knowing fact from fiction when we talk about poison ivy is that people experience its effects, as well as its potential treatments, very differently.

Some people can go years without a reaction after exposure, sometimes even insisting they were *cured* due to multiple exposures, but then be overcome with poisoning years later after one slight contact. There's just no telling how or when this plant will strike over the course of a person's lifetime.

The last basis of considerable confusion lies in the fact that the rest of the animal species, birds, insects, etc., react very differently from humans.

In other words, there is lots of potential for being put off, put out, and put upon by this leafy menace. So read on, and we'll give you everything we know.

But first, take the "test" on the next page to identify any gaps in your own knowledge base.

TEST YOURSELF

Are the following statements
myths or realities?

M	R	Poison ivy/oak/sumac always have 3 leaves.
M	R	You can't get poison ivy/oak/sumac from dead plants.
M	R	You really need to rub it in to get it.
M	R	Poison ivy/oak/sumac vaccines are available.
M	R	Eating its leaves will keep you from getting it.
M	R	Animals can't get poison ivy/oak or sumac.
M	R	Poison ivy/oak/sumac are contagious.
M	R	Poison ivy/oak/sumac are poisonous.

How Did You Do?

1. **SEMI-REALITY: Poison ivy/ oak/sumac always has three leaves.**

   Poison ivy and oak always have the leaves-of-three groupings. Not so for poison sumac (see *Photo Pages* and Chapter III on *Identification* for more detail).

2. **MYTH: Dead plants are not a problem.**

   Poison ivy/oak/sumac oil, *urushiol*, stays active on any surface, including dead plants, for many years, and is just as active in winter as in any other season (though it may be more difficult to see or recognize).

3. **MYTH: You really need to rub it in to get it.**

   Urushiol oil is potent and only one nanogram (one billionth of a gram) is needed to cause a rash.

4. **REALITY: Poison ivy vaccines are available.**

   Scientists have developed a vaccine that can be injected or swallowed, though this vaccine is not often utilized or recommended (for reasons we will explore more thoroughly later).

5. **MYTH: Eating its leaves will keep you from getting it.**

Definitely not a good idea, though we have spoken to a few who swear by this technique as a way to make you immune (see Chapter VII, *Treatment*).

6. **REALITY: Animals can't get poison ivy.**

Animals, except for a few higher primates, are not sensitive to urushiol in the same way that humans are, through skin contact, although they DEFI-NITELY carry it on their fur and can transfer it to humans easily (lots more on this later).

7. **MYTH: Poison ivy is contagious.**

Technically, it's not. You can't get it from some-one by brushing against the rash, but you CAN get it from someone who hasn't washed it off the skin. Experts generally agree that we get it ONLY from contact with the oil itself, not the remaining skin irritation once the oil is gone.

8. **MYTH: Poison ivy is poisonous.**

Technically, poison ivy is not considered a "poison." However, as so many of us know, it often causes a fierce allergic reaction.

Historical Overview: Where does poison ivy come from?

The very first published records of poison ivy in North America date back to the 1600s, when the term "Poison Ivy" was coined by Captain John Smith, in 1609. The name *Poison Ivy* is derived from *urushi*, the Japanese name for lacquer. It is the urushiol (pronounced *oo-roo-shee-ohl*) that gives poison ivy, oak, and sumac their allergic, "poisonous" effects.

Poison ivy is a kind of harmful, climbing vine or shrub in the cashew family. Just think of all the people who are allergic to cashews and other nut oils! It grows plentifully in parts of the United States and southern Canada. Poison ivy specifically, with its three pointed, jagged or rounded leaves, grows in the Eastern, Midwestern and Southern parts of this country. Western poison oak does not appear in the Northeast at all and was, in fact, originally discovered by David Douglas (1799–1834), for whom the Douglas fir was also named, on Vancouver Island, British Columbia.

No one seems to know know where it truly originated, but many of us have noticed ever-widening territorial outgrowths. What could this possibly mean? An environmentalist recently informed me that he believes that poison ivy is indeed "territorial" in this sense: As we continue to develop our lands and remove unwanted growth, the poison ivy continues to spread itself outward to survive and thrive. (Can't you just picture the new thriller, "Night of the Living Poison Ivy?")

Poison ivy usually grows as a vine on tree trunks or straggling over the ground. But the plant often forms upright bushes when it has no convenient support to climb. Both poison oak, which grows in the Pacific Northwest and nearby regions of Canada, and poison sumac, which grows in the Eastern United States, are related species. (See page 14 for *Scientific Classifications.*) There is a type of sumac that is *not* poisonous also. Poison oak and poison sumac are both considered *shrubs*.

For professional workers, such as fire fighters in some states of the United States (California, for example), poison oak reactions, specifically from toxic smoke, are so common that not only are they considered an illness or injury, they are covered by workers compensation insurance and account for an amazingly high percentage of those cases every year.

According to experts at the American Academy of Dermatologists, approximately 85% of the population will develop an allergic reaction when exposed to poison ivy, oak or sumac. Sensitivity seems to develop over several exposures, usually during childhood, and tends to decrease as individuals reach their thirties (although this process has been known to be reversed also).

The plants are certainly a nuisance to people, but compensate, in their unique way, by having considerable wildlife value. The white, waxy berries are a popular food for songbirds during fall migration and in winter when other foods are scarce. Robins, catbirds and grosbeaks enjoy the berries for a gourmet treat, and many different birds feed on insects hiding in the tangled ivy vines. Small mammals and deer graze happily on the poison ivy foliage, twigs and berries.

Goats, sheep, cows, and even horses and pigs love to eat all three plants and are fantastic cleaner-uppers. Just don't give them a hug to thank them for their cleaning skills, because whatever has rubbed onto them can easily rub off onto you.

Allergic reactions to three native American plants—poison ivy, poison oak, and poison sumac, all members of the plant genus *Toxicodendron*, have been sources of chagrin for many centuries. Native Americans made an effort in those days to warn the early settlers about the ill effects of these plants, and Captain John Smith described them in his journal, thus recording the first report of an allergic disease in America. Here are a few statistics that will give you some idea about the plants' demographical effects:

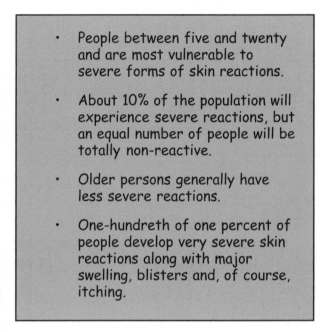

- People between five and twenty and are most vulnerable to severe forms of skin reactions.

- About 10% of the population will experience severe reactions, but an equal number of people will be totally non-reactive.

- Older persons generally have less severe reactions.

- One-hundreth of one percent of people develop very severe skin reactions along with major swelling, blisters and, of course, itching.

Scientific Classification of Plants

Kingdom:	*Plantae*
Division:	*Magnoliophyta*
Class:	*Magnoliopsida*
Order:	*Sapindales*
Family:	*Anacardiaceae*
Genus:	*Toxicodendron*

Species:

Toxicodendron diversilobum
(western poison oak)
Toxicodendron pubscens
(poison oak)
Toxicodendron radicans
(poison ivy)
Toxicodendron rydbergii
(western poison ivy)
Toxicodendron vernicifluum
(Laquer tree)
Toxicodendron vernix
(poison sumac)

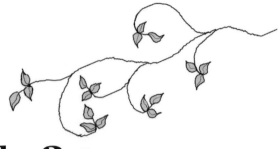

The 3rd Thing to Know

Identifying Poison Ivy, Oak, and Sumac

Know Thine Enemy!

Do all three poison plants look the same? Ben Franklin's adage, *"Leaves of three: Let Them Be!"* is one that still works every time and is a good place to start. We do believe we have occasionally viewed leaves of five woven in among the poison ivy vines, but it may have been sheer paranoia working overtime. Fortunately, the same simple, yet effective, saying works for poison oak too.

Appearance

The compound leaves of poison ivy and oak consist of three pointed leaflets; the middle leaflet has a much longer stalk than the two side ones. The leaflet edges can be *smooth* or *toothed*, also called *notched* or *jagged*. Two of the leaflets form a pair on opposite sides of the leafstalk, while the third stands by itself at the tip of the leafstalk. The leaves vary greatly in size, from 8 to 55 mm in length.

Sumac leaves present in pairs (usually anywhere from 7 to 13) off the primary stalk. All three plants in our poison plant trio change seasonally: they are reddish when they emerge in the spring, turn a shiny green later in spring and through the summer, and become various shades of yellow, orange or red in the autumn.

Early on, small greenish-whitish flowers grow in bunches attached to the main stem close to where each leaf joins it. Later in the season (in late fall, winter and again in early spring), clusters of poisonous berries form. They are whitish, with a waxy look, and often change from white to red. A friend of ours told me that when she and her siblings were young, their mother told them to *"pick the pretty berries"* for a bouquet. Needless to say, the results were not pretty at all.

Location

The three plants in our trio all carry membership in the cashew family (its precise scientific classification *is anacardiaceae*) and, as we indicated earlier, grow abundantly in most parts of the United States and southern Canada (See page 18 for *Demographic Table*). The native plants grow in the woods, fields, in city parks and in gardens. They grow by the ocean side, in sun or shade, and in wet or dry places. They are extremely hardy and fight back any attempts at elimination.

The plants' growth habit depends on where they flourish, resulting in trailing ground cover, freestanding shrubs or vines supported by trees, shrubbery, fences, or other structures. The vines and bark around the vine are particularly noted for their *hairy* nature, seen easily when climbing around the trunk of a tree *(see Photo Pages)*. This attribute can be the final clue that what you're seeing is really poison ivy or oak. And remember, the vine is just as dangerous—that is, it contains just as high levels of urushiol oil—as the leaves and other plant parts.

DEMOGRAPHICS

Plant	Location	Type of Growth
POISON IVY	North, Northeast, South, Southeast, Parts of Southwest, Mountain States, Central States	Vine or shrub, Crawling or climbing; 3-leaf groupings
POISON OAK	Entire West Coast, E. TX, AK, LA, N. FL, NJ, PA, VA, W. VA, NC, SC, GA, AL, MS, AR, OK, TN, OR	Vine or shrub, Crawling or climbing; 3-leaf groupings (most of the time)
POISON SUMAC	Along Mississippi River and all Eastern United States	Shrub; 7 to 13 leaves, in pairs

BELIEVE IT OR NOT!!!

In one reported incident, lacquer from a Chinese jar that may have been buried for centuries caused a poisonous reaction in the people who found it!

And when the Japanese restored the gold leaf on the Golden Temple in Dyoto, they painted urushiol lacquer on it to preserve and maintain the gold's luminous quality. It wouldn't be unreasonable to say that anyone foolish enough to steal from that Temple would be caught "red-handed!"

One really great way to identify whether what you're seeing is oak or ivy is to look at the vines (or stalks) of the plant. If thorns are in evidence, it is NOT either one. Thorns appear on lots of look-alikes, such as berry bushes of all kinds. The leaves of the berry bushes are also kind of fuzzy looking, like a peach. (See Photo Gallery) However, BEWARE, because the poisonous trio often lurks amongst these other plants.

Your Notes Here:

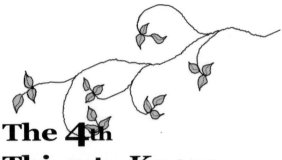

The 4th Thing to Know

Who Gets Poison Ivy, Oak, or Sumac...and Why?

What *is* Poison Ivy...Exactly?

Rashes or conditions due to contact with poison ivy, oak, or sumac are called *rhus dermatitis* which simply means *inflammation of the skin*.

The inflammation is caused by the urushiol oil, the clear, gummy, heavy sap or resin from the plants that is so incredibly reactive that a pinhead amount can cause rashes in hundreds of sensitive people. This fearsome threesome of oily plants is the cause for three of the most common types of allergic *contact dermatitis* in North America.

The oils of the three plants are not identical; however, they are very similar in chemical composition, and most people allergic to one will also react to all three. Many people are unaware that when a person comes in contact for the first time with one of the plants, no visible reaction will occur. In fact, most people will not even realize that they have come in contact with the substance at all.

- At least 80% of the population will develop a skin rash when contacting the leaves of the plant. The severity of the rash varies from person to person.

- Almost all parts of the body are vulnerable to the sticky urushiol, producing the original characteristic linear (line-like) rash (see Photo Pages). Because the urushiol must penetrate the skin to cause a reaction, places where the skin is thick, such as the soles of the feet and the palms of the hands, are "less" sensitive (though it's only a matter of degree) than areas where the skin is thinner. The severity of the reaction also depends on how big a dose of urushiol the person has received.

If a reaction (in the form of a rash) does appear, it may be seven to ten days after the first exposure. Many low-level exposures over a period of years are generally necessary for an individual to reach this level of sensitization, and some people never develop an allergy to poison ivy, oak or sumac plants—*lucky devils.*

What are some of the most common ways of getting poison ivy?

Because urushiol is inside the resin of the plant, rubbing or crushing the stem or a leaf provides sufficient contact for an allergic reaction. Very small amounts of the chemical can provoke a serious reaction in a susceptible person. Here are some typical ways people "catch" poison ivy:

- **Pets**. Your dog or other pet touches other dogs (etc.) who have touched poison ivy, and then you touch your dog, cat, etc.
- **Gardening Supplies**. Gloves are a must! But then, don't forget to wash the gloves every time you use them. Just

tossing them onto a shelf until the next usage isn't good enough, let alone an effective avoidance tactic. And don't forget that dead leaves are still poison ivy leaves, and that the plants have complex root systems under the ground.

- **Sports**. Stray baseballs, hit, thrown or "lost" into areas of brush, are then picked up, held in gloves, and passed from hand to hand. They go directly into cars, then on into homes, etc.

- **Households**. The homes of the "unaware" can be bastions of poison ivy residue. Most people are unconscious about what they might be trucking in on the bottom of their shoes, etc. The plant oil doesn't stay outdoors, but hitches a ride inside on boots, clothes, skin, animals, etc. It then transfers easily to household objects and furniture and to other unsuspecting souls.

The Stuff That Makes Us Itch

Why are people so sensitive to urushiol oil in the first place?

Urushiol oil is very potent. Take a look at these statistics (read 'em and weep):

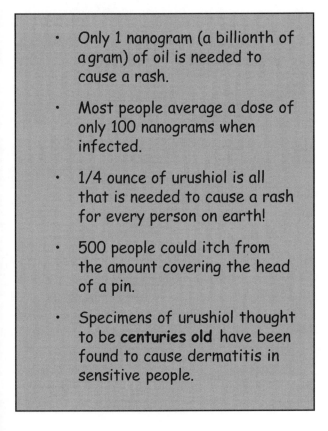

- Only 1 nanogram (a billionth of a gram) of oil is needed to cause a rash.

- Most people average a dose of only 100 nanograms when infected.

- 1/4 ounce of urushiol is all that is needed to cause a rash for every person on earth!

- 500 people could itch from the amount covering the head of a pin.

- Specimens of urushiol thought to be **centuries old** have been found to cause dermatitis in sensitive people.

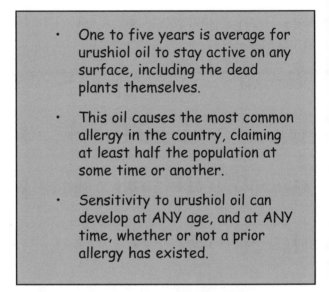

- One to five years is average for urushiol oil to stay active on any surface, including the dead plants themselves.

- This oil causes the most common allergy in the country, claiming at least half the population at some time or another.

- Sensitivity to urushiol oil can develop at ANY age, and at ANY time, whether or not a prior allergy has existed.

Why/How Does the Oil Spread?

Why is it so easy to get poison ivy oil on our skin, our clothes, etc.?

Urushiol oil is easily transferable. Though animals do not contract poison ivy themselves, the oil travels on animal fur without difficulty. It also can be carried in air particles or smoke and on clothes, other plants, etc.

As happened to Randy many years ago, severe cases continue to occur from sap-coated soot in the smoke of burning plants that travels through the air and into mouths, lungs, and throats with potentially fatal consequences.

Immunity

Can you build up an immunity to poison ivy?

Although lots of people can go for long periods of time without a bout of poison ivy, an allergic reaction can reappear at any time without warning. As for building up an immunity to poison plants by eating one leaf a year, here's what one individual had to say: *"My younger sister ate poison ivy to prove that she had developed an immunity to it by eating a couple of leaves every year. This last time she wasn't so lucky. She promptly had a massive reaction, and ended up in the hospital."* Enough said.

Pets and Poison Ivy

Is poison ivy dangerous to my pet?

As those of us know who have sick pets, it's not easy to know the circumstances or the nature of the cause when they become ill. We know they've probably managed to get into something they shouldn't have, but it sure is difficult sometimes to know just what.

In essence, none of the three poison plants, oak, ivy or sumac, affect our pets by allergic reaction through contact with their fur or skin. However, and this is critical, **it is very dangerous for them to ingest. Puppies and kittens are especially susceptible to having strong allergic reactions to its toxicity.**

Again, birds and certain other animals can eat poison ivy berries without any negative repercussions.

Cases have also been reported in people who have used the twigs of the plant for firewood or the vines for Christmas wreaths. Hanging this kind of wreath over a hot hearth can cause considerable damage.

CURIOUS AND *CURIOUSER!*

Recently, Randy developed an allergy to certain nuts, including CASHEWS. Now that we know about poison ivy's close relationship with the cashew family, it all makes sense.

Interesting also is the fact that the seed coats of the plum-sized fruit of Ginkgo trees contain small amounts of urushiol oil. Ginkgo trees were once native only in China, but are now common in almost every city throughout the United States. Although the fruit can be subjected to a detailed process for edibility, many people are still allergic to it.

All these substances that contain the oil cause the same types of reactions when the oil makes contact with the skin. Animals that come in contact with the resin inside the pulp can easily spread it to humans, too, so beware the licks of loving pets.

CONSIDER THIS!

Because urushiol is inside the plant, brushing against an intact plant alone will not cause a reaction. But that's really just about impossible, according to experts, since the plants are so fragile. The stems, leaves, etc., are easily punctured or broken by the wind or animals, and even the tiny holes made by chewing insects can release the oil.

Notes:

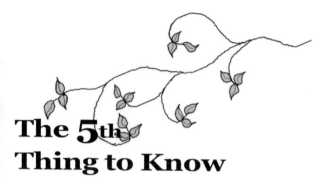

The 5th Thing to Know

The Poison Ivy, Oak, and Sumac Reaction: What Happens?

People Symptoms

Allergic reactions

Approximately 24 to 36 hours after a sensitized person is exposed to the urushiol, an itching rash develops, either with or without blisters. This is what is called a basic *allergic reaction*.

Oil binds to skin

Usually within 15 minutes of contact, the urushiol binds to skin proteins. For those rare people who react after their very first exposure, the rash appears after seven to ten days.

The first physical symptoms

The first symptoms of poisoning from poison ivy, oak, or sumac are severe itching and redness of the skin where it has touched the plant (or other object). This is when the rash appears linear in nature (see *Photo Pages*). Later, the red skin becomes inflamed and blistering of the skin occurs, sometimes along with swelling.

In severe cases, oozing sores develop. After reaching their peak in a few days (usually 7 to 10), the blisters break and the oozing sores begin to crust over and disappear.

Most experts agree that the rash is spread by the poisonous sap, not as the result of contamination from sores!

As mentioned in the last section, poison ivy rash rarely appears on the scalp, palms of the hands or soles of the feet because the skin there is very tough and it is, therefore, more difficult, though still possible, for the oil to penetrate.

When urushiol oil is washed off with lots of water and then soap (such as Fels Naptha, a basic detergent soap), and then liberal amounts of water again *before* the oil has penetrated the skin, a reaction *may often* be prevented.

The blood vessels develop gaps that leak fluid through the skin, causing blisters and oozing. When you use water to help cool down the skin's temperature, the blood vessels constrict, helping to keep them from leaking as much.

Common Questions & Answers

Can I spread it by scratching?

Although some people continue to disagree, we concur with the theory that (1) after the urushiol oil is *fixed* (i.e., has been incorporated through the skin and into the body's cells), it cannot be washed off or transferred to other areas, and (2) it is only when the oil remains on the skin that it is considered prone to spread.

Scratching or oozing blister fluid is not believed to spread the oil to other areas of the body or to other persons. Wounds can become infected, however, and you may make any potential scarring worse. In very extreme cases, excessive fluid may need to be withdrawn by a doctor. Because the course of the reaction is usually 12 to 15 days, two weeks of medication (commonly steroids) is often prescribed.

New lesions that appear a few days after the primary lesions represent less sensitive areas where less antigen was deposited. Again, our experiences have shown that these newer lesions do not represent spreading of the antigen itself.

ALLERGIC REACTIONS

In general, an allergic reaction is a sensitivity or overreaction by the body to a substance that does not cause a problem in "most" people. These substances are called allergens, and include mold spore, dust, food, pollen, etc. Reactions may take many forms: for example, the sneezing and runny nose of hay fever (pollen allergy) or the itching and skin rash of hives (peanut allergy). When these allergic reactions develop within minutes of exposure to an allergen, they are called "immediate hypersensitivity reactions."

Does poison ivy leave scars?

The skin rash from a poison ivy allergy reaction does not ordinarily leave scars unless there is a secondary bacterial infection with deeper skin involvement. This does happen with severe cases of poisoning.

Will I get sick when I get poison ivy?

Symptoms may take as long as two weeks to appear, and sometimes flu-like symptoms, such as headache and fever, also accompany the rash.

Is more oil inside the blisters?

Although this topic is up for considerable discussion, debate, and disagreement among people who can't figure out how their poison ivy, oak or sumac condition seems to "return on its own," sometimes "weeks later," the scientists who study the oil and its effects insist that the blister fluid does not contain active urushiol oil. The appearance of "spread" appears, in actuality, to be a *delayed contact reaction* of oil still on the skin, not oil that exists inside the blisters.

Animal Symptoms

Symptoms of plant poisoning occurring in pets, especially younger animals who are more susceptible, include:

- Difficulty breathing
- Change in pupil size
- Stumbling
- Convulsions
- Unconsciousness
- Vomiting
- Diarrhea
- Nervousness

IMPORTANT INFO!

Using a lawn mower can cause the oil from the plants to become airborne, spreading it all over your lawn and the neighbors' lawn, into your eyes and lungs, onto your clothes, etc. It also has the potential of finding its way—very easily—into your lungs or an animal's lungs, as with burning the leaves and/or entire plants. The oil becomes a gas and is extremely toxic for most people and most pets. So, **BEWARE BURNING BUSHES!**

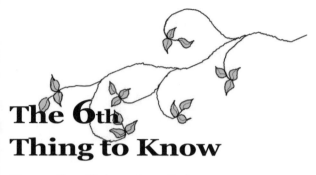

The 6th Thing to Know

Preventing Poison Ivy, Oak, or Sumac

Tests and Vaccines

Dr. William Epstein is the nation's most experienced researcher in the field of poison ivy. He and his colleagues developed a test to determine sensitivity levels to poison ivy. He says it's hard, though, for someone to know for certain how sensitive he or she is because often they haven't experienced a reaction since childhood. Sensitivity can change with time, also, so some people become less sensitive as they age, and others who used to be able to "go swimming" in it can suddenly be severely affected. For example, we've known women who have become allergic when they hit menopause, and men who, for no reason at all, started to experience symptoms suddenly.

Is there a skin test to measure sensitivity?

The skin test itself that researchers developed is similar to the one for tuberculosis exposure, and is no different from other skin tests for other allergies. This test is available at doctors' offices only.

When a doctor needs to confirm suspicions of an allergy, s/he can perform what is called a *patch test*. Because the substance used in the patch test itself may sensitize patients to urushiol, the test is recommended only when necessary for diagnosis, not as a routine procedure. In any case, doctors wait until all active sores have healed because testing can aggravate the condition further.

How is the test done?

Basically, a small drop of diluted urushiol oil is placed on the arm. About 72 hours after a skin test there will be: (1) *nothing*; (2) *a red spot*; (3) *a red spot with swelling and itching*; or (4) *a red spot with blisters*. Pretty simple test, really, but not one most people like to take!

Is there a vaccine against poison ivy?

Scientists have developed a vaccine that can be injected or swallowed. But this is effective **only** if taken before exposure. The poison ivy vaccine is given in injection form once, monthly, for three consecutive months.

People usually experience a temporary, localized heightened sensitivity. Protection against poisoning is neither complete nor permanent; however, there have been reports of milder- or shorter-duration bouts of the rash resulting from receiving this series of vaccinations.

Who can get the vaccine?

Adults and children greater than twelve years of age are eligible to receive vaccination. Children under twelve years of age can only be given this vaccine at the discretion of the physician.

What is the vaccine made of?

The principle, active, toxic ingredient in this vaccine is urushiol, extracted from leaves of poison ivy, oak or sumac. We'd like to remind our readers here that all vaccines utilize other substances in their preparation that can cause reactions themselves. Please check with your health care provider to consider its use.

When can I get the vaccine?

Ideally this vaccine should be given when the plant is still "dormant" during the late winter months. However, it can also be given any other time of the year, *providing you have not been recently exposed and/or do not already have a rash from exposure to poison ivy at the time.*

Avoidance

Unfortunately for all of us, keeping away from poison ivy is not always easy. And avoidance is the only real way to ensure successful prevention.

In lieu of that possibility, however, the best way to avoid the irritating rash is being able to identify the plants in all their iterations (refer to *Identification*, Chapter III).

Avoiding Direct Contact

Direct contact with the plants is the easiest way to contract poison ivy, oak or sumac. After the oil has touched the skin, it usually takes at least a few minutes for it to penetrate and do its damage.

Decontaminating Clothing

You can decontaminate clothing by laundering with soap or detergent. Wear protective gloves (and launder them also—immediately). Any clothing that might have come in contact with the oil should also be washed prior to bringing it indoors or by bringing it indoors wrapped in a sturdy bag, and dumping the whole load directly into the washing machine.

> ALL other items, such as garden tools and hunting or fishing gear, that you use for any purpose in the outdoors, should be washed if they have been in contact with you and/or the plants.

Removing Plants

Efforts have been made to destroy these kinds of plants by uprooting them or by spraying them with chemicals. But poison ivy is so common that these typical methods are not very effective in eliminating them altogether.

The herbicides most commonly used to eradicate poison ivy (which will be explored later in this book), will kill other plants as well. If you don't want to use chemicals, manual removal is always an option and will eventually get rid of the plants, but diligence is key. You have to get every bit of the plants, leaves, vines and roots, or else they will simply sprout again.

The plants should be thrown away according to your municipality's regulations. Although urushiol will break down with composting, the plants must be chopped into small pieces first, which just adds to the time you're exposed to the plant and risk of a rash, so be careful!

One way to avoid regrowth that has been suggested to us, is to lay down a plastic tarp over the area of plants you have sprayed. If you do this over the complete area, you should then be able to lay down a layer of earth or stones so that new growth cannot penetrate.

One landscaper we spoke to said that he was hired to landscape one-half acre of land where a new home had been built. He actually asked the owners if there were any poison ivy plants around. The owners thought not. Unfortunately, though the "top" side of the land was free of any indication that plants flourished there, the dead and decaying leaves were still under the ground as were the roots. Our sad landscaper was covered from head to toe, having taken no real precautions.

The moral? Always take precautions, whether you think it's there or not, and, again, *remember*,

---

Urushiol oil is carried in the smoke and can cause serious lung irritation, lung damage, hospitalization, and even death—for people and their pets alike. So, NEVER, EVER, BURN OR MOW DOWN THE PLANTS!

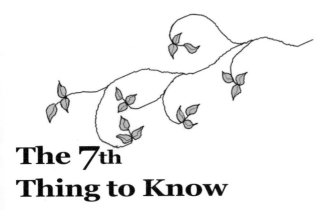

The 7th Thing to Know

Treating Poison Ivy, Oak, and Sumac Conventionally

General Treatments

Wash first and wash well

Start with the basics. As previously mentioned, if you don't cleanse quickly enough, or your skin is so sensitive that cleansing didn't help, redness and swelling will appear in about 12 to 48 hours.

Blisters and itching will certainly follow. The poison ivy reaction can be reduced, however, if you change clothing immediately and wash the exposed skin with water, then soap. If you can wash all the oil off exposed skin within a very short time (5 to 10 minutes), often no reaction will occur at all. Even water from a running stream alone is a very effective cleanser.

Many people swear by *hot water treatments* and *cold water treatments*, more extreme versions of the same process (see Chapter VIII, *Household Treatments*).

Washing infected skin as soon as possible with cold water to minimize the severity of the rash and prevent the spread of the sap to uninfected parts of the body is critical. Unfortunately, however, the skin can absorb the active compounds in the sap very quickly, and once that happens you cannot prevent the onset of symptoms.

Soap and water after water alone is best to continue to remove any sap residue, but this duo can also temporarily remove a naturally protective layer on the skin that helps keep the active compounds from being absorbed through the skin. **So remember...WASH, WASH, WASH! FAST, FAST, FAST!**

Animal Treatments

What do you do if you think your pet has ingested poison ivy or any other poisonous plant?

Immediately (that means before you do anything else!), call your vet or the National Animal Poison Control Center at 1-800-548-2423.

Information to always have on hand

It's always good to have the following information on hand if you can, so that your vet or the Poison Control Center can know as much as possible in order to make decisions about what to do.

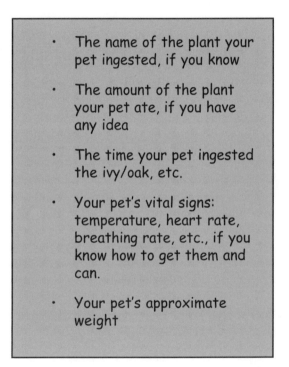

- The name of the plant your pet ingested, if you know

- The amount of the plant your pet ate, if you have any idea

- The time your pet ingested the ivy/oak, etc.

- Your pet's vital signs: temperature, heart rate, breathing rate, etc., if you know how to get them and can.

- Your pet's approximate weight

Naturally, it's best to comfort your pet and make him/her feel secure and head on out to the vet. It's a good idea to take a sample of what your pet ate to the vet with you, if you do in fact know what it is.

If your pet has inhaled the smoke from poison ivy or oak, get the animal to fresh air as quickly as possible!

Should I try to get my pet to vomit if I think s/he has ingested a poisonous plant?

Under rare circumstances, it may be alright to induce vomiting, but you should *always* check with your vet or the Poison Center first. Many times vomiting can make your pet's condition worse; some poisons can cause even more damage on the way back up than they did on the way down.

Never give your pet Syrup of Ipecac (a syrup that automatically produces vomiting) without the vet's okay. Again, sometimes, in the process of vomiting a substance back up into the pet's throat, lungs, digestive track, etc., more damage can be caused.

What's the best way to wash my pet after a romp in the poison ivy?

Who hasn't had a dog or a cat charge off after a skunk or a squirrel? When they finally come back, tail between their legs, they may well be covered with poison ivy residue from plants you've never seen. So don't forgive and forget too soon.

First, wash your pet the same way you would yourself when you've come in contact with poison ivy. Remember: you can't see it and your pets don't tell you, so be preventative.

Start with large volumes of water. Then wash with a mild oil-resistant soap such as Fels Naptha, or a nontoxic, mild laundry detergent. Then wash with lots of water again. Sometimes we add baking soda or hydrogen peroxide if there is a "scent" issue as well. We like to use a hose and try to make it a playful, interactive adventure and, though our dog might disagree with our methods (and may well disagree about the "playful adventure" part), we are at least successful in accomplishing our course of action.

Human Treatments: Conventional

Exterior protective barriers

Unfortunately, we have not personally found any protective barrier that would *totally and consistently* stop poison ivy in its tracks. However, there are a couple of products on the market that we list here that you could try with which some people have indicated good results.

- Barrier creams such as *Ivy Block*, *Multi-shield*, and *Tecnu* (with bentoquantam 5%) can be applied to the skin prior to exposure and will form a protective layer on top of the skin.

- *Ivy Block* is advertised as an "easy to use nonprescription, preexposure lotion. You apply it like sunscreen to all exposed skin. It dries quickly and [it] guards you against the harmful oil in poison ivy [oak]" (From *Ivy Block's* website; refer to References). Lotion should be removed with running water and soap after the risk of exposure has ended.

- *Trental* may decrease the rash somewhat, but is a drug that needs to be taken prior to exposure to the plants, and that can be pretty hard to anticipate and even harder to rely on.

Exterior lotions and creams

Well, if the worst has happened—you have the scourge we call poison ivy—here are some of the best recommended treatments for applying externally to the rash and/or blisters.

Please remember: *We do not advocate for use of any particular product because where one person may swear by the use of one, another person will feel that product is relatively useless.* So, itcher beware. Whatever works, as long as it's safe, use.

- *Tecnu* also makes a skin cleanser, again for use on exposed skin. One workshop participant told me that she uses it over and over immediately after she believes she's been exposed and has not gotten poison ivy.

- If poisoning develops and increases with blisters and red, itching skin, dressings of calamine lotion, *Epsom* salts or bicarbonate of soda can be helpful.

- Nine months pregnant with my first child and 104 degrees outside, I had poison ivy all over my feet. They were red, swollen, burning, and fantastically itchy. The only thing that seemed to relieve the pain was soaking my poor feet in a tub of ice water.

- Cortisone cream is considered by many to be the best treatment. It's recommended to use for at least 2 to 2-1/2 weeks because often the poison ivy lasts that long. Cortisone is said to counteract the growth of white blood cells so there is less inflammation, and allows the system to beat the poison ivy on its own. This treatment often works well in mild-to-moderate cases.

- *Zanfel* Poison Ivy Cream is supposedly a great cure according to *Zanfel's* website information and testimonials. This is an expensive product, but may be well worth trying.

There are a number of topical products that can help dry up the oozing blisters, including:

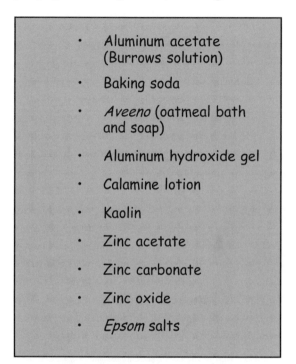

- Aluminum acetate (Burrows solution)
- Baking soda
- *Aveeno* (oatmeal bath and soap)
- Aluminum hydroxide gel
- Calamine lotion
- Kaolin
- Zinc acetate
- Zinc carbonate
- Zinc oxide
- *Epsom* salts

Severe rashes, especially those covering large areas or accompanied by above-normal body temperatures, should always be examined by a health care provider.

Medical treatment, (often in the form of a course of steroids) is most effective if applied/dispensed before the oozing sores appear.

Possible Infection Clues

Any one or more of the following symptoms could signal an infection that may require antibiotic treatment.

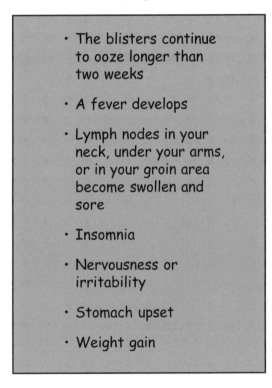

- The blisters continue to ooze longer than two weeks

- A fever develops

- Lymph nodes in your neck, under your arms, or in your groin area become swollen and sore

- Insomnia

- Nervousness or irritability

- Stomach upset

- Weight gain

Possible medical reactions

A health care provider should also be consulted if the medication prescribed for the poison ivy causes any of these side effects:

Internal medicines

Severe reactions can be treated with prescription oral corticosteroids. Some physicians prescribe oral corticosteroids if the rash is on the face and/or genitals, or covers more than 30% of the body.

Some people have even been known to have an allergic reaction that looks like hives when they are on steroids (including yours truly). Be aware and report any skin changes right away.

It is also indicated that this kind of drug must be taken for at least 14 days, and preferably over a three-week period, because shorter courses of treatment will likely cause a rebound with an even more severe rash.

> Again, severe rashes, especially those covering large areas or accompanied by above-normal body temperature should be examined by your health care provider immediately.

PHOTO GALLERY

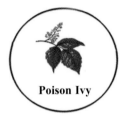

Poison Ivy

Poison ivy, oak, and sumac ALL hold urushiol oil in every part of the plant—stems, vines, leaves, berries, etc. Both ivy and oak leaves are always in groups of three (usually 8 to 55 mm in length).

Poison oak grows in the same types of environments as poison ivy, and is recognizable by the same traits. It is more common to see poison oak, however, growing as a shrub or as ground cover than in the form of climbing vines. One often sees waxy, whitish berries (that also change color) attached to the stem of the plants.

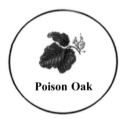

Poison Oak

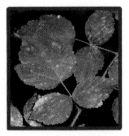

Don't be fooled by harmless plant look-alikes, such as raspberries and strawberries. Notice the much larger third leaf, the telltale thorny stalks, and the fuzzy, peach-like texture of the leaves.

Poison sumac can cause just as ferocious a reaction as ivy and oak, but is very different in appearance. Notice the leaves that shoot off from the stem in pairs of 5, 7, 9, or even 13.

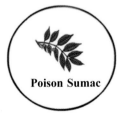

Poison Sumac

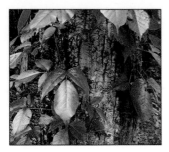

Poison ivy and oak comes in all sizes and shapes. The third larger, middle leaf of the triplet always has the telltale longer stem. Ivy, oak, and sumac carry the toxic urushiol oil in every part of the plant, in every season, dead or alive. Burning or mowing the plants is dangerous because the oil in the smoke or the particles in the air can be inhaled by humans and pets alike. (Examples of poison ivy in the different seasons, top; poison oak, below.)

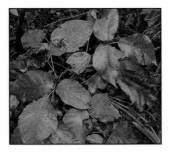

(Photos compliments of Theresa Ford Jonathan Ley, and Betsy and Jim Dunphy)

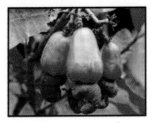

As many people are allergic to nuts, it comes as no surprise that the oil in cashews are related to the urushiol oil found in poison ivy, oak, and sumac.

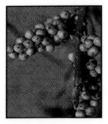

Berry clusters in their full-blown glory (above).

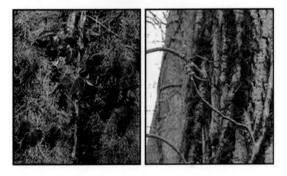

Two excellent examples of poison ivy vines, climbing up and wrapping around these trees. The vines have the signature hairy texture (left) as well as the beginnings of white berry clusters (right). (Photos compliments of Theresa Ford)

Blisters are common, an uncomfortable symptom of an allergic reaction. This ankle rash is recovering from infection (right).

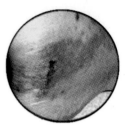

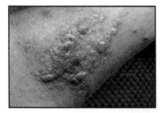

Poison ivy and oak may appear different, but the results are always the same: itching, itching, and more itching...sometimes along with blisters, swelling and pain.

Typical rash on both arms of an unhappy youth.

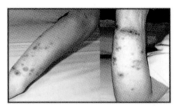

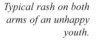

This rash reveals the siganture "linear" pattern (left) along with blistering.

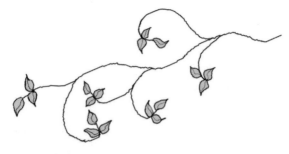

The **8**th Thing to Know

Treating Poison Ivy, Oak, and Sumac with Common Products and Common Sense

"HELP...I'M GOING CRAZY!!!"

It's not uncommon for people to try just about any-thing when they're absolutely crazed with itching and burning and pain.

Have you heard the one about...?

Here are some of the things we know that poison ivy and oak victims have tried. Some of them we have also tried personally, or they have come from our research.

- **Drinking goat's milk.** Well, in fact, it's long been claimed that drinking milk from goats that have grazed on poison ivy/oak/sumac can give immunity. And although it's never been tested, it "may" work (according to Dr. Byers, one of Dr. Epstein's colleagues from the University of California, as of this writing). This may be because goat's milk probably has traces of urushiol oil in it and would be acting similarly to creating a vaccine.

- **Hemorrhoid cream.** One person resorted to this medication, having nothing else on hand. (A common beauty tip in Hollywood for puffy eyes, we can see the correlation!) This cream is made from Tronolane (the active ingredient is pramoxine hydrochloride, 1%), and seemed to help with the tching and swelling and to speed up the drying process. You may not want to go around advertising you're using this particular product, though...

- **Lacquer thinner.** One fellow sufferer soaks lacquer thinner in a rag and then wipes himself down. He says he's been taking this particular course since 1969 and insists it stops the itching and that the rash goes away in a day or two. This kind of effect may be based on the premise that the "poison" is an oil, and the thinner evaporates oil based substances like paints. However, we personally do not feel that paint thinner has qualities that would make it an appropriate option for treating external skin conditions, let alone considering what it could do to our internal systems.

- **Urine.** Here is one idea passed down through three generations. Wipe your own urine on the infected area and let dry. This particular contributor insists the urine dries up the poison and you see results the next day! *He notes one has to use one's own urine for this treatment to be effective.*

- **Gasoline**
- **Honey**
- **Antiperspirant**
- **Skim Milk**

And Now for Plain, Old, Ordinary Common Sense

Tried and true, all-natural treatments are cheap, easy, safe and on our list of favorites by far. Let's start with the *cold water treatment.*

- **Cold water treatment.** Rinse as soon as possible. All our sources agree with this tactic to some degree. Use a LOT of COLD water and quickly or you'll just spread the oil around. Rinse many times because water inactivates the oil. Soap is considered unnecessary by many, although my husband, a Fels Naptha soap advocate, swears by it.

  Don't forget that timing is the main consideration: after being exposed douse yourself immediately with water because the oil usually bonds with skin in as little as 15 minutes or less. Rubbing alcohol is a little more effective initially than water, but the important part is how quickly you rinse the oil off.

- **Hot water treatment.** First, be certain to cleanse the skin BEFORE taking a hot bath or shower because heat releases histamine and that's what causes the itching in the first place. Hot water will cause intense itching as the histamine is released. But, if the heat is gradually increased to the maximum tolerable level and continued, the itching will subside.

Often the hours of relief can help you obtain a much-needed good night's sleep.

- **No treatment.** It's true! In mild cases, the rash, blisters and itch normally disappear in 14 to 20 days at the most without any treatment at all. But few of us can handle the itch and/or resultant blisters, without looking for some relief. In the mildest of cases, wet compresses or soaking in cool to cold water can be effective.

- **Salt water and sun.** If you have the opportunity, many people, including the authors, recommend going down to the ocean to soak the oil away. Randy and I agree that this can relieve the itching as well, after the fact. Taking alternating periods in the ocean and then in the hot sun helps too.

- **Chlorinated water.** Also a common suggestion: hop down to your local swimming pool and play fish for a while. The chlorine can have medicinal value, and there is no risk of spreading the poison ivy to others in the pool.

RANDY & HEIDI'S FAVORITE METHODS

We wash immediately (if not before) using cold water, then Fels Naptha laundry soap, an inexpensive yellow bar of soap found in any supermarket detergent aisle. We take it with us everywhere as a precautionary measure. It seems to remove oils really, really well. It's important to note here once again, however, that some say soap spreads the oil. So, always use water first—it's a sure bet.

We spend as much time as possible at the ocean because salt water seems to be a wonderful cure-all. We soak for 10 minutes, lie in the sun and dry out, and repeat the process as many times as we can.

We also highly recommend a method that we have used for 15 years for all kinds of ailments. This treatment is not "immediate" as is water to try to remove the oil initially, but the most effective cure we've found if, in fact, you're unlucky enough to have the rash already. We go see our physician who is also a traditional, Chinese-trained herbologist. His belief is that there are inherent differences in people who get poison ivy (or other ailments) and those who do not. In the case of poison ivy, this difference lies in how strong and healthy their kidneys are. In this case, people with strong kidneys will be more likely to be able to urinate out the poison from their bodies. Those with weaker kidneys cannot, and the poison eventually releases through their skin.

The individualized herbs we obtain (and then boil and steep and drink) don't usually taste great (in fact they taste abysmal), but help us find relief the fastest and the most effectively. *Well worth the effort.*

And yet some others products:

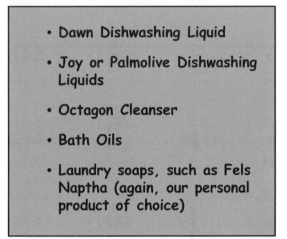

- Dawn Dishwashing Liquid

- Joy or Palmolive Dishwashing Liquids

- Octagon Cleanser

- Bath Oils

- Laundry soaps, such as Fels Naptha (again, our personal product of choice)

These are all good products for ridding the skin, just like your dishes or clothes, of oil. "Plain" soap is not nearly as effective, so try detergents specifically designed to go after oils and greases.

All these great ideas can be added to your list of potential treatments. Some of them we think you'll find *very* interesting.

- Dr. West's Poison Ivy Cleanser
- Inside of a banana peel
- Burts Bees Poison Ivy Soap
- Vinegar
- Rhubarb
- Pepcid AC
- Miracle Whip
- Monistat (vaginal) cream
- Noxema Pads
- Ammonia
- Nail Polish Remover

All of the above mentioned remedies—and many more—have been suggested as "cure-alls" if not simply helpful, but have never been tried by the author. We assume that anything natural (such as milk or honey) could not possibly hurt, but anything you would not ordinarily pour on your skin (such as bleach or gasoline) we would all do well to stay away from altogether.

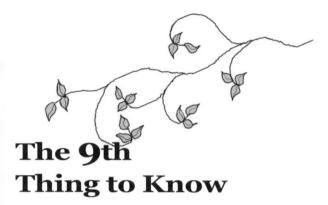

The 9th Thing to Know

Treating Poison Ivy, Oak, and Sumac Homeopathically

Randy and I prefer to use the most basic, or natural, alternatives for treating poison ivy that we can. The following are some of the substances listed by poison ivy sufferers as being the most effective and helpful. Again, we are obligated to note that we have not tested all of the products mentioned here. Please use all/any of them at your discretion.

> • **Goldenseal root powder and aloe vera gel.** Both of these substances are much more commonly used and found as ingredients in drug store products these

days which helps their accessibility. You can make a paste out of goldenseal root powder and the aloe and rub it onto the infected areas. The abrasive quality of the goldenseal can feel great and the mixture will help draw out toxins. The aloe also seems to help to keep the skin from scarring.

- **Dry skin cream with Jewelweed leaves, aloe vera gel and vitamin E.** This method involves blending dry skin cream with crushed Jewelweed leaves, aloe vera gel, vitamin E and vitamin A. Jewelweed is a wild impatiens plant that often grows near poison ivy, a common occurrence that the Native Americans attribute to what the Great Spirit said about "putting the cure next to the cause in nature" (paraphrased liberally).

- **Rat vein tea.** We read about one man whose 88-year-old neighbor swears by this old southern remedy. I don't know where—or if—you can buy rat vein tea, but it is made from the plant which is a member of the wintergreen family, and found in the shade in the woods, blooming from June to August. You never know…if you can find it, it just may work!

- **Touch-Me-Nots.** "Touch-me-not" is simply another name for Jewelweed. For **external** use only, take the stems and flowers and boil them in water. Let it cool and rub it on your skin for instant relief. A woman we know who mixes and prepares her own Jewel Weed-based products even suggests freezing the mixtures for wintertime exposures.

  Of course, out in the wild world, don't hesitate to break open a stem of Jewelweed to rub on your skin—it can be quite serviceable in a pinch.

- **Jewelweed—plain.** For internal use, boiling Jewelweed leaves into a tea for drinking is considered helpful. We have experimented a little with Jewelweed and know it is one of nature's blessings, but our suggestion is to always test a substance such as this externally first before ever trying it internally. Remember, for external use, Jewelweed grows near many poison ivy and related plants. You can often recognize it by its small, delicate, yellow or orange flowers, so it's a great method to try when you're in the great outdoors, especially if you want to use natural substances and/or have nothing else.

- **Minty Lotion soothes itching.** This recipe comes directly from a friend who owns a health food store. She swears by this concoction: Take 1 oz. grindelia oil, 1 tsp. vegetable glycerin, and 5 drops peppermint essential oil. Combine in 2 oz. spray bottle. Shake and apply 4 times per day for relief of itching and pain.

- ***Rhus Toxicodendron* tablets.** These tiny tablets are available at health food stores, and are currently well known for alleviating quite a number of different symptoms associated with allergic rashes, hives, and chicken pox **along with** poison ivy, oak, and sumac, such as itching, redness or swelling.

Rhus "Thox" is also indicated for inflammations of the respiratory passages, gastrointestinal tract, eye, paramnea, headaches, neuralgia, lameness, paralysis, vertigo, periosteum, joints, tendons, and muscles, anxiety and restlessness.

Many people also suggest taking regimens of Rhus Thox to avoid becoming infected in general. Please read up on the suggestions that come with this remedy and/or discuss it wherever you buy this product to learn more about it.

The 10th Thing to Know

Eradicating Poison Ivy, Oak, and Sumac

Natural Methods

Arthur and Elvis were absolutely, hands-down, the best poison ivy eradicators in the business. *Who are they and what's their phone number?* Well, you could try the petting farm, because Elvis and Arthur are goats. **Yes, goats.** Goats, sheep, cows, pigs and even horses not only eat poison ivy/oak/sumac (not to mention your shorts and the side of the house), but *love* to eat poison ivy. Keep a couple of adorable, smart goats and you may keep your poison ivy problem at bay. For those of us who aren't fortunate enough to have goats near by, however, we have to do the next best thing: eliminate it as effectively and as non-toxically as possible.

Getting Rid of It Naturally

Poison ivy is difficult—but not impossible—to eradicate. Of course, the hardest part is trying to avoid poisoning while you're trying to remove it! Always wear protective clothing and try to cover as much of your skin as possible.

The other really positive things about removing poison plants "naturally," is that you won't have any fear about your pets being adversely affected by any chemicals you use, either by rubbing it or eating it. The same goes for your own health and the best interests of our planet.

Repeated cutting

Repeated cutting to the ground will eventually starve out the plant's root system. Cutting with a powered "weed-eater" is NOT a good idea, since it increases the likelihood of spraying the plant oil all over the tool, the user and the area.

Lots of poison ivy climbs high into trees. To kill it, cut the vine six inches above ground level. Then use your choice of product to treat the stump immediately after cutting to kill the roots and prevent sprouting.

Cutting vines to remove small plant growth

Once you have cut the vines at ground level where they have wound up around tree trunks or hedges, remove the smaller plants by pulling with your glove-covered hands, or even with a hoe. Use herbicides of choice on regrowth areas…and just keep pulling.

Pulling and grubbing

As above, pulling and grubbing are effective means of removal, but you need to have close contact with the plants and this kind of treatment will probably need to be repeated more than once.

Chemical Methods

Even though we don't personally like using chemical treatments, from our research very few other types of treatments are as effective in controlling poison ivy, oak and sumac in areas where other plants also grow. The ones we mention here are both *glyphosates* and have been recommended by professional landscapers and gardening experts alike.

- **Round-Up,**
- **Kleen-Up,** and
- **Brush-B-Gon** are...

all absorbed through the leaves and carried throughout the entire plant system. After spraying, leave the plants for several days in order to allow the chemical to be absorbed down through to the root system.

Even people reluctant to use herbicides have indicated that these products really do the job. And with newer products specifically for poison ivy, you don't have to worry about the other plants in the surrounding locale. These products are all fairly expensive.

Remember:

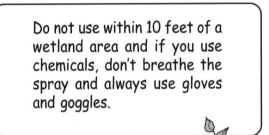

Do not use within 10 feet of a wetland area and if you use chemicals, don't breathe the spray and always use gloves and goggles.

Environmentally Safe Household Methods

Let's talk *good for everyone*. Using what is good for yourself, your family, and the planet simply *works*. These methods simply take common sense and raise it to a whole new level.

- **Removing Single Plants.** To remove single, young plants is possible by grasping them through a plastic garbage bag and pulling up—roots and all. Turn the bag inside-out over the plant and, voila, you're done. You may have some growth return from broken roots, but can get rid of them in the same way if you're vigilant.

- **Salt.** The recommendation to use salt (mixing three pounds of salt with one gallon of soapy water) and spraying the solution on the plants leaves and stems is not recommended as an environmentally healthy method. Although we use salt in our food, the amount we have to use to destroy poison ivy can be more toxic than chemicals, and it does not break down in the environment. Not only that, it can continue to kill anything planted on that spot and leach into the groundwater. So, say "NO" to salt!

- **Removing Large Areas of Growth.** One woman we spoke with told us she eliminated about 1/4 acre of solely poison ivy plants using Ortho's Brush-B-Gon product, saying it was "incredible" when applied with a paint brush to all large old growth stems. It must have been a giant-sized brush!

- **Vinegar.** Well, we saved the best for last. That's right. Last year a relative told me that she had gotten rid of lots of stubborn weeds where she played tennis in places where the plants were coming through the clay of the court. How? **With plain, ordinary, white vinegar.**

My brick walk was forever sprouting weeds of all kinds, so I tried it. And it really works, better than anything else I tried, even the chemical products. And it's extremely affordable. I've been dousing the little bits of poison ivy I've seen around the house and so far we're winning the war.

Vinegar is really the best and the cheapest solution, and the little talked about favorite of garden center staff in-the-know, but it does kill other plants around it, so be careful where you spray it, paint it or pour it on.

ONE FINAL STORY
(SAVING THE BEST FOR LAST)

Randy was living in Oxford, Massachusetts and had a terrible case of poison ivy, one of his last bouts, I am happy to report. In sheer desperation he decided to try to contact the local Nipmuk Indian tribe which has a substantial presence in nearby Webster, MA. He actually ended up talking to the local chief, Chief Wise Owl. Well, to make a long story short, Randy sheepishly posed the following question, "The Native Americans in our old movies are always depicted running around the woods, usually half-naked. How did you guys protect yourselves from getting poison ivy?"

The Chief did not take any offense at the question and, in turn, startled Randy by asking if he knew where the term "red man" came from. Randy said *no,* feeling slightly awkward at the nature of the question.

Chief Wise Owl continued, saying that if the local Natives knew they were going to spend a lot of time in the woods, they would make a mixture of okra and bear grease which they spread over their bodies to cover and protect them. Then, as the sun's rays would hit this mixture, it would both harden the bear grease and turn the okra bright red! This mixture created a protective barrier from poison ivy as well as from most insect bites.

Though okra and bear grease have never been easily available, Randy thanked the Chief, and figured out a way to put the idea to use.

When working outside, he began to cover his face and any other exposed spots with vaseline which seemed to serve the same protective function, though messy for sure.

Chief Wise Owl also (albeit reluctantly, and a little sheepishly himself) suggested that in emergencies another remedy can help (you might recall this particular one we mentioned in Chapter VIII, given to us by a fellow sufferer): Dab your own urine on the poison ivy rash to help it heal more quickly. Again, we have not personally tried this remedy, but under extreme conditions, desperate enough, we just might.

Randy will always be thankful for Chief Wise Owl's willingness to share this ancient Native American wisdom with him.

Your Notes Here:

REFERENCES

Helpful Web Sites

1. www.ivyblock.com (Introduction to plants; ivyblock lotion, etc.)
2. www.zanfel.com (Ivycure@aol.com; information about Zanfel cream product and other poison ivy/oak aspects)
3. www.poison-ivy.org (photo quiz, poster, stories and great pictures of the plants)
4. www.aad.org/pamphlets (American Academy of Dermatologists site; good information)
5. www.ncnatural.com ("Revenge of the Botanicals Close Encounters"—check it out!)
6. www.teclabsinc.com (1-800-ITCHING; from the makers of Tecnu products)
7. www.yourhealth.com (general information about poison ivy, oak, etc.)
8. www.healthy.net/library (HealthWorld on-line emergency and first aid information)
9. www.museum.gov.ns.ca (close-up photos of plants)
10. www.poison-ivy-protection.com (site for *Oral Ivy*, a natural homeopathic poison ivy treatment and pre vention)
11. www.cattail.nu (one of my personal favorites to visit. Theresa Ford has been kind enough to provide some of the excellent photos for this book.

12. www.poisonivy.aesir.com (a site full of information; Jim and Betsy Dunphy also contributed photographs for this book)
13. www.brendanichols.tripod.com/fun/ratsvein.html (for information about rat vein plants)
14. http://www.phlumf.com (site with pictures and words describing this individual's journey on the Pacific West Trail, including details on poison oak. Jonathan Ley was also kind enough to contribute photographs for this book)

RESOURCES

1. American Academy of Allergy, Asthma and Immunology
2. Poison Ivy, Oak & Sumac Information Center, Missouri Department of Conservation, PO Box 1808, Jefferson City, MO 65102-0180
3. Dr. West's Poison Ivy Cleanser: This non-oily spray can be ordered by calling toll-free 1-877-4-DRWEST or (504) 885-3666.

To order copies of these

10 things to know™

books

Poison Ivy, Pets, & People

and

Bees & Other Stinging Insects

Phone orders: please call IPG at 1-800-888-4741,
or visit our website at
www.2lakespublishing.com,
or visit your local bookstore